GALVESTON DIET COOKBOOK FOR MENOPAUSE

Easy-to-make recipes to aid in weight loss and balancing hormones.

+Bonus: 4-weeks fasting schedule & 4-weeks check-in plans.

By. Maria Misner

Disclaimer

This book's content is not meant to be used as medical or health advice; rather, it is meant to be educational and informative only. No medical condition should be diagnosed, treated, or otherwise resolved by using the information. Always with your doctor or other trained health experts before beginning any new medical treatment or condition. The publisher and author disclaim all liability for any particular health requirements that may call for medical care as well as for any harm or unfavorable effects that may arise from any course of action, treatment, application, or preparation taken by anybody who reads this book or uses the information it contains. The references are given purely for informative purposes and do not imply any support for any websites or other sources.

<u>Bonus</u>

4-Week Fasting Schedule for Beginners from beginners to advanced.
The 4-weeks check-in plan is at the ultimate chapter to help you track your progress.

Week 1: Introduction

Day 1-3:

  - Fasting Window: 12 hours (e.g., 8 PM - 8 AM)

  - Eating Window: 12 hours (e.g., 8 AM - 8 PM)

Day 4-7:

  - Fasting Window: 13 hours (e.g., 8 PM - 9 AM)

- Eating Window: 11 hours (e.g., 9 AM - 8 PM)

Week 2: Gentle Extension
Day 8-10:
  - Fasting Window: 14 hours (e.g., 8 PM - 10 AM)
  - Eating Window: 10 hours (e.g., 10 AM - 8 PM)
Day 11-14:
  - Fasting Window: 15 hours (e.g., 8 PM - 11 AM)
  - Eating Window: 9 hours (e.g., 11 AM - 8 PM)

Week 3: Intermediate Fasting
Day 15-17:
  - Fasting Window: 16 hours (e.g., 8 PM - 12 PM)
  - Eating Window: 8 hours (e.g., 12 PM - 8 PM)

Day 18-21:
   - Fasting Window: 17 hours (e.g., 8 PM - 1 PM)
   - Eating Window: 7 hours (e.g., 1 PM - 8 PM)

Week 4: Sustainable Routine
Day 22-24:
   - Fasting Window: 18 hours (e.g., 8 PM - 2 PM)
   - Eating Window: 6 hours (e.g., 2 PM - 8 PM)
Day 25-28:
   - Fasting Window: 16 hours (e.g., 8 PM - 12 PM)
   - Eating Window: 8 hours (e.g., 12 PM - 8 PM)

Quick Tips:
1. Start Slow: Don't rush the process. Listen to your body and make gradual changes.

2. Stay Hydrated: Drink plenty of water.

3. Nutritious Meals: Focus on balanced meals with adequate protein, healthy fats, and fiber to keep you full and energized, which are going to be discussed later in the book.

4.Avoid Perfection: If you occasionally break your fast early, don't be discouraged. Progress is more important than perfection.

About The Author

Maria Misner is a loving mother, an outspoken supporter of wellbeing and self-care. Maria has devoted her life to discovering and disseminating the keys to leading a healthy and flourishing existence. She has a strong interest in holistic health, exercise, and nutrition. Her personal experiences and her desire to feel and look her best at every stage of life led her to embark on her health quest.

Maria understands the particular difficulties and rewards associated with striking a balance between her own health and her family life. Because her observations and useful counsel are based on her experience, readers from a variety of backgrounds may relate to and use it.

Maria is passionate about leading a healthy lifestyle that goes beyond appearances; she feels that genuine wellbeing can only be attained by taking care of one's mind, body, and soul. This mentality is reflected in her approach to the Galveston Diet for menopause, which gives readers a thorough manual for navigating this momentous life change with grace and vigor.

In this book, Maria blends her passion for cooking with her understanding of the Galveston Diet's tenets to provide scrumptious and nourishing dishes that are tailored to the requirements of menopausal women. Her cookbook is more than simply a list of recipes; it's evidence of her dedication to promoting the health and happiness of others.

Table Of Contents

Introduction

My menopause and me

I had to navigate the difficult menopausal transition, just like many other women. I had a plethora of symptoms, including constant exhaustion, mood changes, heat flashes, and weight gain. I had the impression that I was losing control over my physical appearance.

I started looking into symptom management techniques because I was determined to find a solution. I found the Galveston Diet at that point. I made the decision to try it. The initial weeks had a steep learning curve.

After a few months, I observed a striking change. Hot flashes subsided, my attitude steadied, and the obstinate weight started to peel away. It was the first time in years that I felt refreshed, in better health, and more attuned to my body. Motivated by my personal experience, I made the decision to disseminate my insights and understanding via this cookbook.

In addition to giving me back control over my health throughout menopause, this diet rekindled my interest in cooking and leading a healthy lifestyle.

An Overview of the Galveston Diet Theory.

The Galveston Diet is a novel dietary strategy created to specifically target the health requirements of women going through menopause.

It is a well-rounded approach designed to assist women going through menopause in managing their weight, achieving optimal health, and lessening the intensity of menopausal symptoms via mindful eating and lifestyle changes.

Including full, nutrient-dense foods that promote hormonal health is a fundamental component of this diet. Essential vitamins, minerals, and antioxidants may be obtained from a range of fruits and vegetables, lean meats, and healthy fats. This method aids in lowering inflammation and promoting metabolic health, all of which are essential for controlling weight and energy levels throughout menopause.

Part 1:
The Pledge: Foundations and Preparation

Chapter 1. Overview of Menopause:

Explanation of hormonal changes during menopause and their effects on the body.

Menopause, which normally happens between the ages of 45 and 55, is a normal biological process that signals the end of a woman's reproductive years. Significant hormonal changes accompany this shift, chief among them being the ovaries' decreased synthesis of progesterone and estrogen.

Many biological processes, such as controlling the menstrual cycle, preserving bone mass, and impacting mood and mental abilities, depend on estrogen. Women may have a variety of symptoms when their estrogen levels fall. Common vasomotor symptoms like night sweats and hot flashes are brought on by abnormalities in the hypothalamus, which controls body temperature. Decreased estrogen also has an impact on the vaginal lining, which can cause atrophy, pain, and dryness.

Menopause also causes a reduction in progesterone, which controls the menstrual cycle and primes the uterus for conception. Before menstruation completely stops, irregular periods may result from this hormone's decrease.

Reduced estrogen causes an acceleration of the loss of bone density, raising the risk of osteoporosis and fractures. Weight increase and changes in the distribution of fat, particularly around the belly, might result from metabolic alterations. Hormonal changes can have an effect on mental health by exacerbating anxiety, despair, and mood swings.

Another side effect that is made worse by hot flashes and nocturnal sweats is disturbed sleep. Variations in blood artery function and cholesterol levels can impair cardiovascular health and increase the risk of heart disease.

With any luck, this clarifies the definition of menopause as well as the ramifications of the hormone changes that occur throughout it.

Chapter 2: Weight Management: Insights into why weight gain occurs during menopause and strategies to combat it.

Now, Let's examine why weight changes throughout menopause.

Gaining weight during menopause is a prevalent worry that has several related causes. Hormonal changes, namely the decrease in estrogen levels, are the main cause. Estrogen, as previously mentioned, regulates body weight and metabolism. Reduced levels might cause metabolism to slow down, which can result in weight gain even in cases when food choices stay the same.

Additionally, alterations in body composition are a result of aging itself. Age-related decreases in lean muscle mass can lead to a reduction in the number of calories expended at rest since muscle burns more calories than fat. Sometimes, this makes gaining weight simpler.

Variations in the distribution of fat are another cause. Abdominal fat is frequently the first area to develop after menopause, replacing fat that was more likely to be deposited in the hips and thighs during the reproductive years. Higher health risks, such as diabetes and cardiovascular disease, are linked to this visceral fat.

A big part is also played by lifestyle variables. In midlife, many women see changes in their diets and levels of exercise. Stress, sleep deprivation, and hectic schedules can result in poor food choices and decreased physical activity, which can accelerate weight gain.

Benefits of the Galveston Diet Approach

The Galveston Diet method navigates the difficulties of menopause and offers several advantages.

One of the main advantages is the decrease in inflammation. Chronic inflammation, which is connected to a number of menopausal symptoms and long-term health problems, is reduced by this diet. Decreased risk of chronic illnesses, better cardiovascular health, and less joint problems can all result from reduced inflammation.

This method's promotion of metabolic flexibility and assistance with weight management is another pillar.

It raises general energy levels, increases insulin sensitivity, and helps regulate blood sugar levels. For menopausal women, who frequently battle with weight gain and energy swings, this can be very helpful.

It promotes the intake of lean proteins and healthy fats, which strengthen muscle mass and increase satiety. Additionally aids in preserving a healthy weight and lowers the chance of developing metabolic syndrome.

Overall, by making thoughtful dietary and lifestyle changes, this method provides menopausal women with a well-rounded, scientifically supported plan to help them reach optimal health, control their weight, and lessen the intensity of menopausal symptoms.

Part 2: The Lifestyle

Chapter 3: Anti-inflammatory Nutrition Guide:

Anti-Inflammatory Foods & Detailed list of foods that reduce inflammation.

Though the primary goal of this book is to teach us how to create foods that fit the Galveston diet, which is effective for hormone imbalances and menopause.

On the other hand, anti-inflammatory foods are essential for improving general health and lowering the risk of chronic inflammation-related disorders. These foods are often high in vitamins, minerals, antioxidants, and phytonutrients, which support the body's defenses against oxidative stress and inflammation at the cellular level.

By lowering the synthesis of pro-inflammatory chemicals, healthy fats assist in balancing the body's inflammatory processes.

Legumes and whole grains include complex carbs and fiber that help maintain stable blood sugar levels and promote a healthy gut microbiota, which in turn reduces inflammation.

Many spices and plants, including curcumin and gingerol, have been shown to have anti-inflammatory properties.

All things considered, including a range of these anti-inflammatory foods in a balanced diet will boost immunity, encourage wellbeing, and perhaps lower the chance of developing long-term inflammatory diseases.

Foods to Avoid:
Explanation of foods that promote inflammation

In order to decrease or prevent inflammation, I'm going to share with you some foods that cause it before we go on to the next part.

Reduce or avoid processed foods that are heavy in bad fats and refined sugars. Although it may be challenging, you must complete the task. These consist of sweets, sugary snacks, and meals that include trans fats, which can cause weight gain and inflammation.

Because highly processed carbs can cause blood sugar levels to jump and hormonal balance to be upset, foods like white bread, pastries, and sugary cereals should also be avoided.

Moreover, meals rich in sodium, such processed meats and salty snacks, can aggravate symptoms like bloating and discomfort by causing water retention.

Since they might cause hormone swings and interfere with sleep patterns, caffeine and alcohol should be used in moderation or completely avoided.

By being aware of and steering clear of certain foods and drinks, one can enhance hormonal health, better control inflammation, and enhance general wellbeing throughout menopause.

Foods That Reduce Inflammation & Foods to be Avoided-Or reduced

The lists includes;

1. Fatty Fish
   - Salmon

- Mackerel
- Sardines
- Tuna

2. Fruits
- Berries (strawberries, blueberries, raspberries)
- Oranges
- Cherries
- Grapes

3. Vegetables
- Leafy greens (spinach, kale, collards)
- Broccoli
- Brussels sprouts
- Cauliflower
- Bell peppers

4. Nuts and Seeds
- Almonds
- Walnuts

- Chia seeds
- Flaxseeds

5. Healthy Oils
   - Extra virgin olive oil
   - Avocado oil

6. Whole Grains
   - Brown rice
   - Quinoa
   - Oats
   - Whole wheat

7. Legumes
   - Lentils
   - Chickpeas
   - Black beans
   - Kidney beans

8. Spices and Herbs
   - Turmeric

- Ginger
- Garlic
- Cinnamon

9. Tea
- Green tea
- Black tea

10. Fermented Foods
- Yogurt (with live cultures)
- Kefir
- Sauerkraut
- Kimchi

Foods to Avoid

1.Refined Carbohydrates
- White bread
- Pastries
- Sugary cereals
- White rice

2. Fried Foods
   - French fries
   - Fried chicken
   - Doughnuts

3. Sugary Beverages
   - Soda
   - Sweetened coffee drinks
   - Energy drinks

4. Processed Meats
   - Bacon
   - Sausages
   - Hot dogs
   - Deli meats

5. Excessive Alcohol
   - Beer
   - Spirits
   - Cocktails

6. Trans Fats
   - Margarine
   - Hydrogenated oils
   - Processed snacks (chips, crackers)

7. High Fructose Corn Syrup
   - Many packaged snacks
   - Sweetened yogurts
   - Some salad dressings

8. Excessive Salt
   - Packaged soups
   - Canned vegetables
   - Salty snacks

9. Red and Processed Meat
   - Beef
   - Pork
   - Lamb

10. Artificial Additives
    - Food dyes
    - Artificial sweeteners
    - Preservatives

Chapter 4: Incorporating Periodic Fasting:

Explanation of how periodic fasting aids in weight management and reduces inflammation.

Using the 16/8 approach, I started periodic fasting by eating between noon and 8 PM. During the eating window, I concentrated on eating full, nutrient-dense meals including whole grains, lean meats, healthy fats, and an abundance of veggies. I noticed that my cravings for unhealthy snacks decreased and that I had more energy during the day.

I lost a lot of weight within a few months, especially around my stomach. My clothing fit better, and I had a more self-assured, upbeat feeling.

My own experience demonstrates the advantages of periodic fasting for reducing inflammation and managing weight.

Weight Management with Periodic Fasting

Cycling between eating and fasting intervals, which can last anywhere from a few hours to many days, is known as periodic fasting. The most popular approaches are the Eat-Stop-Eat technique (24-hour fasts once or twice a week), the 5:2 strategy (eating normally for five days and reducing calories for two non-consecutive days), and the 16/8 method (16 hours of fasting and an 8-hour eating window).

The lowering of the eating window, which in turn causes a natural decrease in calorie intake, is one of the main ways that periodic fasting helps with weight management. You may reduce your calorie intake without necessarily keeping track of them if you restrict the times you eat. A calorie deficit is necessary in order to lose weight.

periodic fasting also affects hormones that are essential for controlling weight. Insulin levels decrease during fasting, which promotes fat burning. The body can more efficiently use fat that has been stored as energy when insulin levels are lower. Additionally, norepinephrine, a hormone that speeds up metabolism and helps the body burn more calories, is released in greater amounts during a fast.

Human growth hormone (HGH), which assists in fat burning and muscle preservation, is also produced in greater quantities while fasting. Increased levels of HGH during fasting can help with fat loss and lean muscle maintenance by improving overall body composition.

**Getting Started:
Tips for beginners on how to ease into
periodic fasting.**

Though it may be made easier, periodic fasting may be challenging. A few first actions are as follows:

1. Start Gradually: Set up a 12-hour window for eating and fasting at first. One hour should be added to the fast every few days until you get to a 16/8 schedule.

2. Remain Hydrated: When fasting, make sure to consume lots of water, herbal teas, or black coffee. Maintaining hydration promotes general health and aids in controlling appetite.

3. Consume Foods High in Nutrients: Throughout your eating windows, concentrate on eating entire, nutrient-dense meals like fruits, vegetables, lean meats, whole grains, and healthy fats to keep you fed and satisfied.

4. Listen to Your Body: Observe your feelings. If you feel lightheaded, extremely hungry, or exhausted, change your meal schedule or see a doctor.

5. Stay Busy: During times of fasting, divert your attention from hunger by partaking in hobbies, exercises, or other activities.

6. Eat Balanced Meals: To sustain energy levels and stave off cravings, make sure your meals are well-balanced with a decent combination of protein, healthy fats, and carbs.

7. Be Consistent: To aid your body in adjusting to the new habit, adhere as closely as possible to the fasting plan you have set.

You can more easily and successfully transition into periodic fasting by using the advice in this article.

Periodic Fasting and Reducing Inflammation

Although the body naturally responds to injury or infection with inflammation, persistent inflammation can cause a number of health problems, including as diabetes, heart disease, and autoimmune diseases. It has been demonstrated that periodic fasting lowers inflammatory indicators, which has several positive health effects.

periodic fasting decreases inflammation through a process called autophagy, which is the body's way of removing damaged cells and replacing them with new ones. Autophagy is triggered by fasting and aids in the elimination of cellular waste and damaged proteins that may exacerbate inflammation. This cellular purging not only lowers inflammation but also enhances lifespan and general health.

At the cellular level, periodic fasting influences inflammatory pathways as well. According to studies, fasting can lower the amount of pro-inflammatory cytokines—signaling molecules that encourage inflammation—that are produced. Fasting helps to reduce the body's overall inflammatory response by reducing these cytokines.

periodic fasting also enhances gut health, since inflammation and gut health are strongly related. Inflammation is largely regulated by the gut microbiome, and fasting can support a balanced population of beneficial gut bacteria. Leaky gut syndrome is less likely in those with healthy guts.

Part 3: Plan All Together: Recipes and Meal Plans

Chapter 5: Meal Plans

Creating meal planning can help you maintain a balanced, nutrient-dense diet and make eating easier. Emphasizing whole, unprocessed meals that promote hormone balance and general health is essential.

I'm going to walk you through these meal plans, which are meant to be flexible and accommodating to different tastes and lifestyles. This will make it easier to stick to the plan and enjoy the process of improving your health.

Healthy Breakfasts for Hormones

1. Greek Yogurt with Berries and Nuts

Ingredients:
- 1 cup (245g) of plain Greek yogurt
- 1/2 cup (75g) of mixed berries (e.g., strawberries, blueberries, raspberries)
- 2 tablespoons (14g) of mixed nuts (e.g., almonds, walnuts, cashews)
- 1 teaspoon (7g) of honey (optional)

Nutritional Information

Without Honey:
- Calories: 255
- Protein: 26.5g
- Total Fat: 8.7g
- Saturated Fat: 1g
- Carbohydrates: 19g
- Fiber: 3.5g
- Sugars: 15g

With Honey:
- Calories: 276
- Protein: 26.5g
- Total Fat: 8.7g
- Saturated Fat: 1g
- Carbohydrates: 25g
- Fiber: 3.5g
- Sugars: 21g

To prepare the yogurt, scoop it into a dish.
Add Berries: Sprinkle some mixed berries over the yogurt.
Sprinkle the nuts on top of the berries to add them.
Optional Sweetener: You may optionally top with cinnamon or honey.
Gently stir or blend.
Savor your food!

2. Avocado Toast with Eggs

Most of the lipids in avocados and olive oil are monounsaturated fats, which are good for hormone balance and heart health. These good fats have the potential to lower inflammation, which is especially advantageous during menopause.

Although the egg in this dish contains some saturated fats, they are still within moderation for a diet that is balanced.

Ingredients:
- 1 slice of whole grain bread (28g)
- 1/3 medium avocado (50g)
- 2 large egg whites (66g)
- Salt and pepper to taste

Nutritional Information
- Calories: 184
- Protein: 11.2g
- Total Fat: 8g
- Saturated Fat: 1.2g
- Carbohydrates: 16.6g
- Fiber: 5g
- Sugars: 2.6g

Guide:

Toast Bread: Cook the bread slice according to your preference.

Avocado Preparation: Scoop the avocado into a bowl and mash it with a fork while the bread is toasting. Add pepper and salt for seasoning.

Egg Cooking: You can cook the egg anyway you like it—fried, poached, or scrambled.

Put Toast Together: Toast the bread and then spread the mashed avocado on it.

Put an Egg in It: Top the avocado toast with the fried egg.

Optional Toppings: Sprinkle with red pepper flakes or drizzle with olive oil(little) if desired.

Enjoy: Serve immediately and enjoy!

3. Smoothie Bowl

A high protein content is ensured by the use of protein powder, which is crucial for maintaining muscle mass and feeling full.

Ingredients:
- 1/2 cup (120ml) almond milk (unsweetened)
- 1/2 banana (about 60g)
- 1/2 cup (75g) mixed berries (e.g., strawberries, blueberries, raspberries)
- 1/4 avocado (about 50g)
- 1 scoop (30g) protein powder (plant-based or whey)
- 1 tablespoon (10g) chia seeds
- 1/4 cup (30g) granola (optional)
- Toppings: fresh fruit, coconut flakes, nuts, seeds (optional)

Nutritional Information

Without Granola:

- Calories: 358
- Protein: 24.6g
- Total Fat: 14.6g
- Saturated Fat: 1.9g
- Carbohydrates: 33g
- Fiber: 12.8g
- Sugars: 13g

With Granola:
- Calories: 508
- Protein: 27.6g
- Total Fat: 20.6g
- Saturated Fat: 2.4g
- Carbohydrates: 54g
- Fiber: 15.8g
- Sugars: 21g

Instructions:

Mix well. Basis: Put the milk, banana, mixed berries, avocado, and protein powder (if using) into a blender. Process till smooth.

Transfer to a bowl: Fill a bowl with the smoothie mixture.Include toppings:
Add your preferred fresh fruit, nuts, seeds, or granola on top.
Have fun: Enjoy and serve right now!

4. Oatmeal with Flax Seeds and Fresh Fruit

Dietary fiber, which is important for healthy digestion and blood sugar regulation, is mostly found in oats, flax seeds, and fresh fruit.

Ingredients:
- 1/2 cup (40g) old-fashioned rolled oats
- 1 cup (240ml) water or unsweetened almond milk
- 1 tablespoon (7g) ground flax seeds

- 1/2 cup (75g) mixed fresh fruit (e.g., berries, apple slices, banana slices)
- Optional: a drizzle of honey or maple syrup (1 teaspoon, 7g)

Nutritional Information

Using Water and Without Honey/Maple Syrup:
- Calories: 217
- Protein: 6.8g
- Total Fat: 6.2g
- Saturated Fat: 0.8g
- Carbohydrates: 36g
- Fiber: 8g
- Sugars: 6g

Using Unsweetened Almond Milk and Without Honey/Maple Syrup:
- Calories: 247
- Protein: 7.8g

- Total Fat: 8.7g
- Saturated Fat: 0.8g
- Carbohydrates: 37.5g
- Fiber: 8g
- Sugars: 6g

Using Water and With Honey/Maple Syrup:
- Calories: 238
- Protein: 6.8g
- Total Fat: 6.2g
- Saturated Fat: 0.8g
- Carbohydrates: 42g
- Fiber: 8g
- Sugars: 12g

Using Unsweetened Almond Milk and With Honey/Maple Syrup:
- Calories: 268
- Protein: 7.8g
- Total Fat: 8.7g
- Saturated Fat: 0.8g

- Carbohydrates: 43.5g
- Fiber: 8g
- Sugars: 12g

Instructions:

Cook the Oats: Put the rolled oats and water (or almond milk) in a medium pot. Heat to a boil on a medium setting.

Simmer: After bringing to a boil, turn down the heat to low and simmer, stirring now and again, until the oats are tender and have soaked up most of the liquid, about 5 to 7 minutes.

Add Flax Seeds: Stir in the ground flax seeds and simmer for a further minute to ensure they are well incorporated.

Serve: Remove the saucepan from the heat. Transfer the oatmeal to a bowl.

Top with Fruit: Add the mixed fresh fruit on top of the oatmeal. You can use a variety of fruits based on your preference or what's in season.

Optional Sweetener: If desired, drizzle with honey or maple syrup for added sweetness.

Enjoy: Mix together if you like, or enjoy the layers separately!

5. Chia Pudding

Ingredients:
- 1/4 cup (40g) chia seeds
- 1 cup (240ml) unsweetened almond milk
- 1 tablespoon (15g) maple syrup or honey (optional)
- 1/2 teaspoon vanilla extract (optional)
- Toppings: fresh fruit, nuts, seeds, or granola (optional)

Nutritional Information (Without Toppings)

Without Maple Syrup:
- Calories: 230
- Protein: 7g
- Total Fat: 14.5g
- Saturated Fat: 1g
- Carbohydrates: 19.5g
- Fiber: 15g
- Sugars: 0g

With Maple Syrup:
- Calories: 282
- Protein: 7g
- Total Fat: 14.5g
- Saturated Fat: 1g
- Carbohydrates: 33g
- Fiber: 15g
- Sugars: 13.5g

Instructions:

Mix Ingredients: Combine the almond milk, chia seeds, vanilla essence, and maple syrup (or honey) in a jar or mixing dish. Mix well to blend.

Mix Well: To keep the chia seeds from clumping, let the mixture sit for a few minutes before stirring it again.

 Place a lid on the bowl or jar and place it in the refrigerator for a minimum of four hours or overnight. As the liquid is absorbed by the chia seeds, a pudding-like texture is produced.

Verify Consistency: Examine the consistency upon refrigeration. To get the right thickness, whisk in a bit extra almond milk if it's too thick.

Derve: Ladle into dishes or jars of the chia pudding. Add your preferred fresh fruit, nuts, seeds, or granola on top.

Enjoy: Serve immediately or store in the refrigerator for up to 3-4 days for a quick, nutritious snack or breakfast.

Enjoy!

Lunches and Light Meals

1. Quinoa Salad with Chickpeas and Vegetables

Ingredients:
- 1 cup quinoa
- 2 cups water
- 1 can (15 oz) chickpeas, drained and rinsed
- 1 cup cherry tomatoes, halved
- 1 cucumber, diced
- 1/4 cup red onion, finely chopped
- 1/4 cup chopped parsley
- 2 tablespoons olive oil
- 1 tablespoon lemon juice
- Salt and pepper to taste

Preparation:

1. Give the quinoa a good rinse in cold water. Heat the water in a medium-sized saucepan until it boils.

2. After adding the quinoa, lower the heat to low, cover, and simmer until the water is absorbed, about 15 minutes.

3. Use a fork to fluff the quinoa and let it to cool.

4. Combine the chilled quinoa, chickpeas, cucumber, red onion, cherry tomatoes, and parsley in a big bowl.

5. Combine the olive oil, lemon juice, salt, and pepper in a small bowl. Drizzle the salad with the dressing and mix well.

2. Grilled Chicken and Veggie Wrap

Ingredients:
- 1 large whole-grain tortilla
- 1 grilled chicken breast, sliced

- 1/2 avocado, sliced
- 1/2 cup shredded carrots
- 1/2 cup baby spinach
- 1/4 cup hummus
- Salt and pepper to taste

Preparation :
1. Place the tortilla flat and evenly cover it with hummus.
2. Arrange the shredded carrots, avocado, baby spinach, and chicken slices on top.
3. Add pepper and salt for seasoning.
4. Tightly roll the tortilla, cut it in half, and proceed to serve.

3. Lentil Soup

Ingredients:
- 1 cup dried lentils, rinsed
- 4 cups vegetable broth

- 1 onion, chopped
- 2 carrots, diced
- 2 celery stalks, diced
- 3 cloves garlic, minced
- 1 can (14.5 oz) diced tomatoes
- 1 teaspoon cumin
- 1 teaspoon paprika
- Salt and pepper to taste
- 2 tablespoons olive oil

Preparation:

1. Heat the olive oil in a big saucepan over medium heat.

2. Add the onion, carrots, and celery; simmer for about 5 minutes, or until softened.

3. Cook for a further minute after adding the paprika, cumin, and garlic.

4. Include the chopped tomatoes, vegetable broth, and lentils.

5. After bringing to a boil, lower the heat, and cook the lentils until they are soft, about 30 minutes.

6. For better taste, add salt and pepper for seasoning.

4. Stuffed Bell Peppers

Ingredients:
- 4 large bell peppers, tops cut off and seeds removed
- 1 cup cooked brown rice
- 1 can (15 oz) black beans, drained and rinsed
- 1 cup corn kernels
- 1 cup diced tomatoes
- 1/2 cup chopped cilantro
- 1 teaspoon cumin
- 1 teaspoon chili powder
- Salt and pepper to taste

- 1/2 cup shredded cheese (optional)

Preparation:

1. Turn the oven on to 375°F, (190°C).

2. Transfer the cooked brown rice, black beans, corn, chopped tomatoes, cumin, chili powder, cilantro, and salt and pepper into a big bowl.

3. Stuff the mixture inside the bell peppers and put them on a baking tray.

4. Top the filled peppers with the shredded cheese, if using.

5. Bake the peppers for 30 minutes with a foil cover on, then take the foil off and continue baking for another 10 minutes, or until they are soft.

5. Shrimp and Avocado Salad

Ingredients:

- 1 lb cooked shrimp, peeled and deveined
- 2 avocados, diced
- 1 cup cherry tomatoes, halved
- 1/4 cup red onion, finely chopped
- 1/4 cup chopped cilantro
- 2 tablespoons olive oil
- 1 tablespoon lime juice
- Salt and pepper to taste

Preparation:

1. Put the cooked shrimp, chopped avocados, cherry tomatoes, red onion, and cilantro in a big bowl.

2. Combine the olive oil, lime juice, salt, and pepper in a small bowl.

3. Drizzle the salad with the dressing and gently toss to mix.

4. Present right away.

Dinners to Support Hormones

1. Baked Salmon with Asparagus

Ingredients:
- 4 salmon filets (about 6 oz each)
- 1 bunch asparagus, trimmed
- 2 tablespoons olive oil
- 2 cloves garlic, minced
- 1 lemon, sliced
- Salt and pepper to taste

Preparation:
1.Set the oven's temperature to 400°F, (200°C).
2. Arrange the salmon filets on a parchment paper-lined baking sheet.
3. Position the asparagus in relation to the salmon.

4. Cover the salmon and asparagus with a drizzle of olive oil.

5. Top with a sprinkle of salt, pepper, and chopped garlic.

6. Place slices of lemon on top of the salmon filets.

7. Bake for 15 to 20 minutes, or until the asparagus is soft and the salmon is cooked through.

2. Turkey and Vegetable Stir-Fry

Ingredients:
- 1 lb ground turkey
- 2 cups broccoli florets
- 1 red bell pepper, sliced
- 1 carrot, julienned
- 2 tablespoons soy sauce (or tamari for gluten-free)
- 1 tablespoon sesame oil

- 2 cloves garlic, minced
- 1 teaspoon grated ginger
- 2 green onions, chopped

Preparation:

1. Heat the sesame oil in a big pan or wok over medium-high heat.

2. Add the ground turkey and, using a spoon to break it up, heat until browned.

3. Cook for a further minute after adding the ginger and garlic.

4. Include the carrot, bell pepper, and broccoli. Sauté the veggies for five to seven minutes, or until they are soft.

5. Cook for an additional two minutes after adding the soy sauce.

6. Before serving, sprinkle chopped green onions over top.

3. Quinoa Stuffed Bell Peppers

Ingredients:
- 4 large bell peppers, tops cut off and seeds removed
- 1 cup cooked quinoa
- 1 can (15 oz) black beans, drained and rinsed
- 1 cup corn kernels
- 1 cup diced tomatoes
- 1/2 cup chopped cilantro
- 1 teaspoon cumin
- 1 teaspoon chili powder
- Salt and pepper to taste

Preparation :
1. Turn the oven on to 375°F (190°C).
2. Combine the cooked quinoa, chopped tomatoes, black beans, corn, cilantro,

cumin, chili powder, salt, and pepper in a big bowl.

3. Stuff the mixture inside the bell peppers and put them on a baking tray.

4. Bake the peppers for 30 minutes with a foil cover on, then take the foil off and bake for a further 10 minutes, or until they are soft.

4. Zucchini Noodles with Pesto and Chicken

Ingredients:
- 2 large zucchinis, spiralized into noodles
- 2 cooked chicken breasts, sliced
- 1/2 cup cherry tomatoes, halved
- 1/4 cup homemade or store-bought pesto
- 1 tablespoon olive oil
- Salt and pepper to taste

Preparation:

1. In a big pan over medium heat, warm the olive oil.

2. When the zucchini noodles are somewhat cooked, add them and sauté for two to three minutes.

3. Cook for a further two minutes after adding the cut chicken and cherry tomatoes.

4. Turn off the heat and toss in the pesto, stirring to coat everything thoroughly.

5. Before serving, add salt and pepper to taste.

5. Lentil and Sweet Potato Curry

Ingredients:
- 1 cup dried lentils, rinsed
- 1 large sweet potato, peeled and diced
- 1 onion, chopped

- 2 cloves garlic, minced
- 1 tablespoon curry powder
- 1 teaspoon ground turmeric
- 1 can (14.5 oz) diced tomatoes
- 1 can (14 oz) coconut milk
- 2 cups vegetable broth
- 2 tablespoons olive oil
- Salt and pepper to taste
- Fresh cilantro for garnish

Preparation :

1. Heat the olive oil in a big saucepan over medium heat.

2. Add the onion and simmer for approximately 5 minutes, or until softened.

3. Cook for a further minute after adding the turmeric, curry powder, and garlic.

4. Include the sweet potato, chopped tomatoes, lentils, vegetable broth, and coconut milk.

5. After bringing to a boil, lower the heat, and simmer until the sweet potato and lentils are soft, 25 to 30 minutes.

6. To taste, add salt and pepper for seasoning.

7. Before serving, garnish with fresh cilantro.

Homemade Snacks and Desserts for Balance.

1. Cucumber and Tomato Salad

Ingredients:
- 1 cucumber, diced
- 1 cup cherry tomatoes, halved
- 1 tablespoon balsamic vinegar
- Salt and pepper to taste

Guide:
1. Put the chopped cucumber and cherry tomatoes, cut in half, in a bowl.
2. Add a balsamic vinegar drizzle and season with pepper and salt.
3. Gently toss and serve right away.

2. Celery Sticks with Salsa

Ingredients:
- 4 celery stalks, cut into sticks
- 1/2 cup salsa

Guide:
1. Arrange celery sticks on a plate.
2. Serve with salsa for dipping.

3. Air-Popped Popcorn

Ingredients:
- 1/2 cup popcorn kernels
- Salt to taste

Guide:
1. Pop the popcorn using an air popper in accordance with the manufacturer's directions.

2. Season with salt and serve right away.

4. Carrot and Bell Pepper Sticks

Ingredients:
- 2 carrots, cut into sticks
- 1 bell pepper, cut into sticks

Guide:
1. Slice the bell pepper and carrots into sticks.
2. You may eat them as a crunchy snack by themselves or with a little dip.

5. Frozen Grapes

Ingredients:
- 1 cup seedless grapes

Guide:

1. Wash and dry the grapes.

2. Arrange them on a baking sheet in a single layer, then freeze for one to two hours.

3. Eat straight from the freezer as a cool snack.

These snacks are easy to make, low in fat, and a fantastic way to keep a balanced diet going.

Chapter 6:

Shopping Lists And Pantry Essentials

Maintaining a balanced diet requires having a well-stocked pantry, particularly when emphasizing hormonal health. Making a thorough shopping list may make dinner preparation easier and guarantee you have everything you need on hand. Incorporate a range of complete meals, including whole grains, lean meats, healthy fats, and an abundance of fresh produce. Keeping your pantry stocked with essential culinary supplies, herbs, and spices will help you make healthier meals that taste better. This method not only helps you achieve your nutritional objectives, but it also inspires culinary inventiveness.

Weekly Grocery Lists and Essentials for the Pantry for Simple Meal Planning

Take a look at the following pre-made shopping lists to help you cook meals more quickly and make sure you have everything you need for balanced meals. The list includes:

Proteins
- Chicken breasts (2 lbs)
- Salmon filets (1 lb)
- Canned chickpeas (2 cans)
- Eggs (1 dozen)
- Greek yogurt (32 oz)

Grains
- Quinoa (1 lb)
- Brown rice (1 lb)
- Rolled oats (1 lb)

- Whole-grain tortillas (1 package)

Vegetables
- Spinach (1 bag)
- Bell peppers (3, assorted colors)
- Broccoli (1 head)
- Carrots (1 bag)
- Zucchini (2)

Fruits
- Apples (4)
- Bananas (6)
- Mixed berries (frozen or fresh, 1 lb)
- Avocados (2)

Healthy Fats
- Olive oil (1 bottle)
- Almonds (1 lb)
- Natural nut butter (1 jar)

Condiments and Spices

- Balsamic vinegar (1 bottle)
- Soy sauce (1 bottle)
- Ground cumin (1 jar)
- Garlic powder (1 jar)
- Black pepper (1 jar)

Sweeteners
    - Honey or maple syrup
    - Coconut sugar

Snacks
    - Air-popped popcorn
    - Dark chocolate (70% cocoa or higher)
    - Whole-grain crackers

Herbs and Spices
    - Ground cumin
    - Turmeric
    - Paprika
    - Garlic powder
    - Dried herbs (oregano, basil, thyme)

Miscellaneous
- Granola (1 bag)
- Chia seeds (1 bag)
- Salsa (1 jar)

You can make a variety of meals throughout the week to support your health goals and reduce stress in the kitchen by keeping these essentials on hand. on keep meals interesting and new, you may modify the list according on what's in season or your own tastes.

Chapter 7:

Tips For Long-term Success

It takes constant work and awareness to achieve long-term health and wellness, particularly in terms of hormone balance.

I want to talk about how I've changed on my path and how you can too by establishing reasonable objectives. I went about goal-setting, and you may modify these techniques to suit your particular way of living.

I set attainable, quantifiable objectives that encourage incremental rather than radical improvements. This strategy encourages long-lasting behaviors. The objectives and actions consist of:

1. Determine Your Reasoning

It's critical to know why you want to accomplish a goal. Effectively controlling the symptoms of menopause was important to me. I was motivated to take action because I wanted to feel more balanced and invigorated.

2. Adopt the SMART Structure

I started by using the SMART guidelines:

-Specific: I put a concrete aim in place of a general one, such as "eat healthier," by saying, "I will include a serving of leafy greens in my lunch three times a week."

Measurable: I put a number on my objectives. I set a goal to work out for thirty minutes three times a week so I could readily monitor my progress.

- Achievable: Understanding my limitations, I concentrated on doable objectives like cooking two meals at home a week.

-Relevant: I matched my objectives with my medical requirements. Including meals high in phytoestrogens was very helpful for controlling hormone fluctuations.

   - Time-bound: I set deadlines for myself. For example, I aimed to complete my meal prep every Sunday to set up a successful week ahead.

3. Break Down Bigger Objectives: I divided my larger goals, like reducing weight, into smaller ones. My goal was to lose 1 pound a week by changing the amount I ate and progressively increasing the amount of exercise I did.

4. Remain Adaptable: Unexpected events might occur in life. When my first fitness regimen got hard, I adjusted by taking shorter at-home exercises or going for longer walks during the day to make sure I was still moving but not too busy.

5. Put the Emphasis on Habit-Building: I discovered that it's better to put the development of habits ahead of results. I made a commitment to mindful eating, which improved my pleasure of meals in addition to assisting with weight control.

6. Frequent Check-Ins: I planned reviews for once a week to evaluate my development. This kept me motivated by enabling me to recognize and appreciate little victories, like always adding more veggies to my meals.

I discovered that by customizing these techniques, creating attainable objectives also became entertaining. I urge you to modify these techniques to fit your unique path, enabling you to attain long-term health and wellbeing.

Chapter 8: Check-In Plans: Bonus

4-Week Check-In Plan

Few aims of this plan are:

1. Consistency: Make a habit of daily journaling at the same time each day.
2. Honesty: Be honest with yourself about your successes and challenges.
4. Adjustments: Be flexible and willing to adjust your plan as needed.

Week 1: Getting Started
Focus: Establishing routines and initial adjustments.

Checklist:
1. Daily Journal:
   - Record fasting and eating times.
   - Note meals and snacks.
   - Track hydration (water, herbal teas, etc.).

2. Physical Well-being:

  - Energy levels (morning, afternoon, evening).
  - Sleep quality and duration.
  - Any hunger or cravings.

3. Emotional Well-being:
  - Mood and stress levels.
  - Motivation and any challenges faced.

Weekly Reflection:
- What worked well this week?
- What were the biggest challenges?
- Adjustments needed for next week?

Action Steps for Week 2:
- Make small adjustments based on reflections (e.g., meal timing, food choices).
- Set a goal for Week 2 (e.g., extending fasting window by 1 hour).

Week 2: Building Momentum

Focus: Extending fasting windows and refining dietary choices.

Checklist:
1. Daily Journal:
   - Continue tracking fasting/eating times, meals, and hydration.
   - Note any changes in appetite and energy.

2. Physical Well-being:
   - Changes in energy and sleep.
   - Any physical symptoms (e.g., headaches, digestive changes).

3. Emotional Well-being:
   - Mood stability and stress management.
   - Motivation and support from family/friends.

Weekly Reflection:
- Progress on Week 1 goals.
- New observations about eating patterns or energy levels.
- Adjustments needed for next week?

Action Steps for Week 3:
- Gradually extend fasting windows if comfortable.
- Focus on incorporating more nutrient-dense foods.

Week 3: Deepening the Routine
Focus: Maintaining longer fasting windows and optimizing nutrition.

Checklist:
1. Daily Journal:
    - Continue detailed tracking (fasting/eating, meals, hydration).

- Note any significant changes in appetite or cravings.

2. Physical Well-being:
   - Overall energy and sleep patterns.
   - Any new physical symptoms or improvements.

3. Emotional Well-being:
   - Changes in mood and stress levels.
   - Any motivational dips or boosts.

Weekly Reflection:
- Success in extending fasting windows.
- Challenges faced and how they were managed.
- Adjustments needed for next week?

Action Steps for Week 4:
- Fine-tune fasting and eating windows for sustainability.

- Set a goal for maintaining or slightly modifying fasting schedule.

Week 4: Establishing Long-Term Habits
Focus: Final adjustments and setting up for long-term success.

Checklist:
1. Daily Journal:
   - Track final week's fasting/eating, meals, and hydration.
   - Reflect on overall progress and remaining challenges.

2. Physical Well-being:
   - Final review of energy levels and sleep quality.
   - Physical changes noted (e.g., weight, body composition).

3. Emotional Well-being:

- Overall mood and stress assessment.
- Long-term motivation and support plans.

Weekly Reflection:
- Summary of progress over 4 weeks.
- Key learnings and major challenges.
- Satisfaction with the current fasting/eating schedule.

Action Steps Moving Forward:
- Set long-term goals for maintaining or adjusting fasting routines.
- Plan for continued tracking and reflection (e.g., monthly check-ins).
- Identify resources for ongoing support (e.g., community groups, further reading).

This check-in plan helps you stay engaged and reflect your progress, ensuring that, you can make informed adjustments to

your fasting and dietary habits as you
follow the Galveston Diet Cookbook for
Menopause.

Conclusion

As we come to an end, I hope that this book has given you insightful knowledge and useful tools to assist your health and wellbeing at this life-changing stage. Menopause navigation can be difficult, but with the appropriate strategy, symptoms can be efficiently managed, a healthy weight can be maintained, and general vigor can be enhanced.

In this book, the significance of anti-inflammatory foods, macronutrient balance, and mindful eating techniques customized for menopausal women is emphasized. Whole, nutrient-dense meals, lean proteins, healthy fats, and an assortment of fruits and vegetables can help to improve metabolic health, lower inflammation, and promote hormonal balance.

A major theme in this book is periodic fasting, which helps you manage your weight and increases metabolic flexibility while giving your body time to relax and heal. By promoting a healthy connection with food, self-awareness, and mindful eating practices, this all-encompassing strategy gives you the capacity to take charge of your health.

To make your trip easier and more pleasurable, we have included helpful meal planning, delectable recipes, and necessary pantry essentials throughout this book. Long-term success depends on establishing reasonable, attainable objectives and upholding consistency, flexibility, and adaptability.

Recall that this is a sustained lifestyle shift rather than just a short-term diet. Honor your accomplishments, remain dedicated to your objectives, and practice self-compassion. Every step you take toward improving your health is a constant process.

Ask For Review

I appreciate that you have selected "Galveston Diet Cookbook for Menopause." It is my genuine hope that this book has given you useful knowledge and useful methods to improve your health and well-being at this important stage of life. Your opinions are very valuable to me and to other readers who might find your expertise helpful in the future.

I would appreciate it if you could take a few minutes to provide a review if you found this book to be informative, inspirational, or enjoyable. Your opinions and life experiences can inspire others to pursue better health and assist them in making well-informed decisions.

To help you with your evaluation, consider these questions:
What aspect of this book did you find most inspirational or useful?
- How has using the recipes or information changed your day-to-day routine?
-Are there any particular passages or advice that caught your attention?

-Would you suggest this book to a friend or family member going through menopause? Why?

We value your candid criticism, whether it takes the form of a few sentences or a thorough analysis. Your aid and advice are much appreciated in expanding the book's audience and helping more people use it.

I appreciate you taking the time to participate in this adventure. I hope you stay well and have more success.

Warm regards,

Maria Misner.